DIABETES DIET COOKBOOK FOR SENIORS OVER 50

Delicious and nutritious low-carb and low-sugar recipes for diabetics

Dr. Mary D. Cook

Text Copyright© 2024 by Dr. Mary D. Cook

TABLE OF CONTENTS

OTHER BOOKS BY THE AUTHOR

1. OSTEOPOROSIS DIET COOKBOOK FOR SENIORS

CLICK HERE TO GET YOUR COPY NOW!!!

2. THE ULTIMATE OSTEOPOROSIS DIET COOKBOOK FOR WOMEN

CLICK HERE TO GET YOUR COPY NOW!!!

3. THE ULTIMATE GASTRIC SLEEVE BARIATRIC COOKBOOK

CLICK HERE TO GET YOUR COPY!!!

4. PESCATARIAN DIET COOKBOOK FOR DIABETICS

CLICK HER TO GET YOUR COPY NOW!!!

5. MEDITERRANEAN DIET COOKBOOK FOR RHEUMATOID ARTHRITIS

CLICK HERE TO GET YOUR COPY NOW!!!

5. OSTEOARTHRITIS DIET COOKBOOK

CLICK HERE TO GET YOUR COPY NOW!!!

INTRODUCTION

Welcome to the Diabetes Diet Cookbook for Seniors Over 50! I'm thrilled to share with you the culmination of my years of experience as a nutritionist, **Dr. Mary D. Cook**. Throughout my career, I've been dedicated to helping individuals, especially seniors, manage their health through the power of nutrition. This cookbook is a testament to that dedication, designed specifically for seniors over 50 who are living with diabetes.

My journey into the world of nutrition began with a passion to make a difference in people's lives. One such life-changing encounter was with my dear friend, Amira. Amira and I had been friends for decades, sharing laughter, stories, and, unfortunately, health struggles. Amira was diagnosed with diabetes in her early 60s, and like many facing this diagnosis, she felt overwhelmed and uncertain about how to manage it effectively.

Seeing her struggle, I knew I had to do something to help. With my background in nutrition, I set out to find a solution that would not only help Amira manage her diabetes but also improve her overall health and well-being.

Together, we embarked on a journey of discovery, exploring the transformative power of food as medicine.

What transpired over the following months was nothing short of miraculous. Through a combination of education, support, and delicious, nutritious meals, Amira's health began to improve. Her blood sugar levels stabilized, and she experienced a newfound sense of vitality and energy. But perhaps most importantly, she regained control over her health and her life.

Amira's story is just one example of the profound impact that proper nutrition can have on managing diabetes. It's a testament to the fact that food is not just fuel for our bodies; it's medicine. And as we age, it becomes increasingly important to nourish our bodies with the nutrients they need to thrive.

In this cookbook, you'll find a treasure trove of recipes designed specifically with seniors in mind. Each recipe is carefully crafted to be low in carbohydrates and sugar, making them suitable for individuals managing diabetes. But beyond that, they're also bursting with flavor, ensuring that you never have to sacrifice taste for health.

From hearty breakfasts to satisfying dinners and everything in between, these recipes are sure to delight your taste buds while nourishing your body from the inside out. But this cookbook is more than just a collection of recipes; it's a guide to living your best life, even in the face of a chronic illness like diabetes.

So join me on this journey to better health and discover the joy of delicious, nutritious meals that can help you manage diabetes and enhance your overall well-being. Together, we can take control of our health and embrace a future filled with vitality, energy, and good food. Let's get cooking!

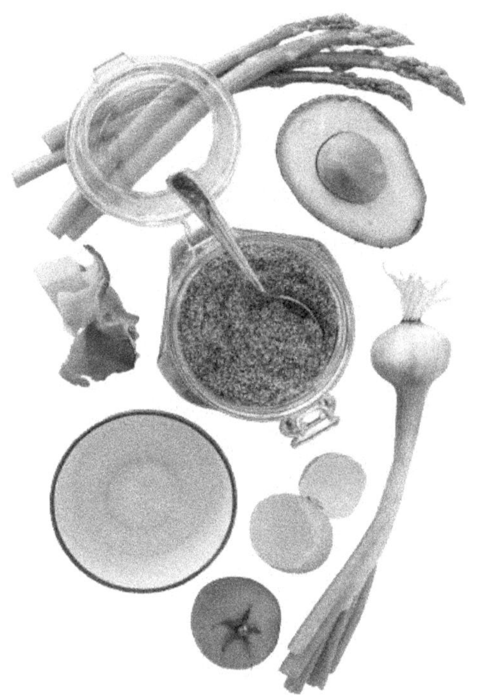

PART ONE

Understanding Diabetes:

Diabetes is a chronic metabolic disorder characterized by elevated blood sugar levels, which result from either the body's inability to produce enough insulin or its inability to effectively use the insulin it produces. Insulin is a hormone produced by the pancreas that helps regulate blood sugar levels and allows glucose to enter cells, where it is used for energy. When this process is impaired, it can lead to various health complications.

Types of Diabetes:

There are several types of diabetes, each with its own causes, symptoms, and treatment approaches. The main types of diabetes include:

1. **Type 1 Diabetes:** This type of diabetes is an autoimmune condition in which the body's immune system mistakenly attacks and destroys the insulin-producing cells in the pancreas. As a result, the body produces little to no insulin. Type 1 diabetes typically develops in childhood or adolescence, although it can occur at any age.

Individuals with type 1 diabetes require lifelong insulin therapy to manage their blood sugar levels.

2. Type 2 Diabetes: Type 2 diabetes is the most common form of diabetes, accounting for the majority of cases worldwide. It occurs when the body becomes resistant to insulin or when the pancreas fails to produce enough insulin to meet the body's needs. Type 2 diabetes is often associated with lifestyle factors such as obesity, physical inactivity, and poor diet. It typically develops in adulthood, although it is increasingly being diagnosed in children and adolescents due to rising rates of obesity.

3. Gestational Diabetes: Gestational diabetes occurs during pregnancy when the body cannot produce enough insulin to meet the increased demands of pregnancy. It usually develops around the 24th to 28th week of pregnancy and resolves after childbirth. However, women who develop gestational diabetes are at an increased risk of developing type 2 diabetes later in life.

4. Other Types of Diabetes: There are also other less common types of diabetes, including monogenic diabetes (caused by a mutation in a single gene) and secondary diabetes (caused by certain medications, diseases, or conditions).

Causes of Diabetes:

The exact causes of diabetes vary depending on the type of diabetes:

- **Type 1 Diabetes:** The exact cause of type 1 diabetes is not fully understood, but it is believed to involve a combination of genetic predisposition and environmental factors. It is thought that viral infections or exposure to certain toxins may trigger an autoimmune response that leads to the destruction of insulin-producing cells in the pancreas.

- **Type 2 Diabetes:** Type 2 diabetes is primarily caused by insulin resistance, which occurs when the body's cells become less responsive to insulin. This can be influenced by a variety of factors, including genetics, obesity, physical inactivity, poor diet (high in processed foods, sugars, and unhealthy fats), and aging.

- **Gestational Diabetes:** The exact cause of gestational diabetes is not well understood, but it is believed to be related to hormonal changes and insulin resistance that occur during pregnancy.

Women who are overweight, older, or have a family history of diabetes are at increased risk of developing gestational diabetes.

Symptoms of Diabetes:

The symptoms of diabetes can vary depending on the type and severity of the condition. Common symptoms of diabetes include:

- **Frequent Urination:** Excess glucose in the blood can cause the kidneys to work harder to filter and absorb the sugar, leading to increased urination.

- **Excessive Thirst:** Dehydration resulting from increased urination can cause excessive thirst.

- **Unexplained Weight Loss:** In type 1 diabetes, the body may begin to break down fat and muscle tissue for energy when it cannot access glucose from the bloodstream.

- **Increased Hunger:** Without adequate insulin to transport glucose into cells, the body may signal hunger to compensate for the lack of energy.

- **Fatigue:** Insufficient glucose uptake by cells can lead to fatigue and weakness.

- **Blurred Vision:** High blood sugar levels can cause fluid to be pulled from the lenses of the eyes, affecting vision.

- **Slow Healing of Wounds:** High blood sugar levels can impair the body's ability to heal wounds and fight infections.

- **Frequent Infections:** Individuals with diabetes are more susceptible to infections, particularly yeast infections (such as thrush) and urinary tract infections.

It's important to note that some people with type 2 diabetes may not experience any symptoms, especially in the early stages of the disease. This is why regular screening and monitoring of blood sugar levels are crucial for early detection and management of diabetes.

Preventive Measures for Diabetes:

While some risk factors for diabetes, such as age and genetics, cannot be changed, there are several lifestyle modifications and preventive measures that can help reduce the risk of developing type 2 diabetes and manage existing diabetes effectively:

1. **Maintain a Healthy Weight:** Excess body weight, particularly abdominal fat, increases the risk of insulin resistance and type 2 diabetes. Losing weight through a combination of healthy eating and regular physical activity can help improve insulin sensitivity and reduce the risk of diabetes.

2. **Adopt a Healthy Diet:** A well-balanced diet that is rich in fruits, vegetables, whole grains, lean proteins, and healthy fats can help regulate blood sugar levels and promote overall health. Limiting the intake of processed foods, sugary beverages, and foods high in unhealthy fats and refined carbohydrates is important for diabetes prevention.

3. **Engage in Regular Physical Activity:** Exercise helps improve insulin sensitivity, lower blood sugar levels, and maintain a healthy weight. Aim for at least 150 minutes of moderate-intensity aerobic exercise, such as brisk walking or cycling, per week, along with muscle-strengthening activities on two or more days per week.

4. **Monitor Blood Sugar Levels:** Regular monitoring of blood sugar levels is essential for individuals with diabetes to ensure that they are within target ranges. This can help identify any fluctuations in blood sugar levels and guide adjustments to medication, diet, and exercise as needed.

5. **Manage Stress:** Chronic stress can increase the risk of type 2 diabetes by raising blood sugar levels and promoting unhealthy behaviors such as overeating or physical inactivity. Practicing stress-reduction techniques such as meditation, deep breathing exercises, or yoga can help manage stress and improve overall well-being.

6. **Quit Smoking:** Smoking is associated with an increased risk of type 2 diabetes and can worsen diabetes-related complications such as heart disease and nerve damage. Quitting smoking can significantly reduce the risk of developing diabetes and improve overall health.

7. **Limit Alcohol Consumption:** Excessive alcohol consumption can contribute to weight gain, increase blood sugar levels, and impair insulin sensitivity. Limit alcohol intake to moderate levels (up to one drink per day for women and up to two drinks per day for men) or avoid it altogether to reduce the risk of diabetes.

8. **Get Regular Check-ups:** Regular medical check-ups, including screenings for diabetes and related complications, are important for early detection and management of the disease. This includes monitoring blood pressure, cholesterol levels, kidney function, and eye health.

Diabetes is a complex and chronic metabolic disorder that requires careful management to prevent complications and improve quality of life. By understanding the different types of diabetes, their causes, symptoms, and preventive measures, you can take proactive steps to reduce their risk of developing diabetes and lead healthier lives. Through a combination of healthy lifestyle choices, regular monitoring, and medical management, diabetes can be effectively managed, allowing individuals to live fulfilling and active lives.

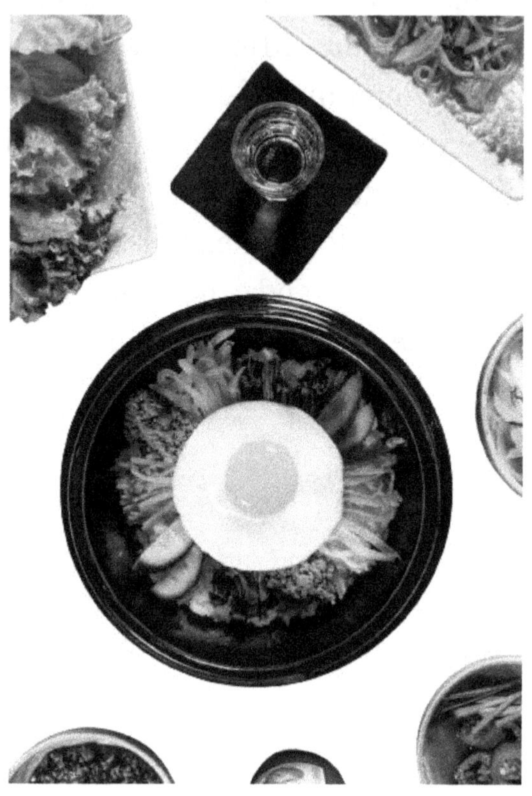

PART TWO:

Achieving optimum health while managing diabetes requires careful attention to diet, especially for seniors over 50. A balanced and nutritious diet can help control blood sugar levels, prevent complications, and enhance overall well-being. Here's a guide to the foods to eat and avoid on a diabetes diet for seniors over 50:

Foods to Eat:

Non-Starchy Vegetables: Fill your plate with a variety of colorful non-starchy vegetables such as leafy greens, broccoli, cauliflower, peppers, and carrots. These vegetables are low in carbohydrates and calories but rich in fiber, vitamins, and minerals, making them an essential part of a diabetes-friendly diet.

Whole Grains: Choose whole grains over refined grains to increase fiber intake and improve blood sugar control. Opt for whole wheat bread, brown rice, quinoa, oats, barley, and bulgur. Whole grains provide sustained energy and help stabilize blood sugar levels.

Lean Proteins: Include lean sources of protein in your meals to help maintain muscle mass and keep you feeling full and satisfied. Good options include skinless poultry, fish, tofu, beans, lentils, and low-fat dairy products. Limit red meat and processed meats, which may increase the risk of heart disease and other complications.

Healthy Fats: Incorporate healthy fats into your diet to support heart health and improve insulin sensitivity. Choose sources of unsaturated fats such as olive oil, avocado, nuts, seeds, and fatty fish like salmon and mackerel. These fats help reduce inflammation and promote overall health.

Fruits: Enjoy fruits in moderation as part of a balanced diet. Opt for fresh or frozen fruits with lower glycemic indexes such as berries, apples, pears, and citrus fruits. These fruits provide vitamins, minerals, and antioxidants without causing rapid spikes in blood sugar levels.

Dairy: Include low-fat or non-fat dairy products in your diet for calcium, vitamin D, and protein. Choose plain yogurt, skim milk, and reduced-fat cheese over full-fat options to reduce saturated fat intake and support heart health.

Nuts and Seeds: Snack on small portions of nuts and seeds for a satisfying crunch and a dose of healthy fats, protein, and fiber. Almonds, walnuts, pistachios, chia seeds, and flaxseeds are excellent choices for seniors with diabetes.

Herbs and Spices: Enhance the flavor of your meals with herbs and spices instead of salt, sugar, or high-calorie condiments. Experiment with herbs like basil, cilantro, rosemary, and spices such as cinnamon, turmeric, and ginger to add depth and complexity to your dishes.

Foods to Avoid:

Processed Foods: Minimize your intake of processed and packaged foods that are high in refined carbohydrates, added sugars, unhealthy fats, and sodium. These foods can cause rapid spikes in blood sugar levels and contribute to weight gain and inflammation.

Sugary Beverages: Avoid sugary drinks such as soda, fruit juices, sweetened teas, and energy drinks, as they provide empty calories and can lead to fluctuations in blood sugar levels.

Opt for water, herbal tea, or sparkling water with a splash of lemon or lime instead.

Sweets and Desserts: Limit consumption of sweets, candies, pastries, cakes, cookies, and other sugary treats, as they can cause blood sugar levels to soar. If you have a sweet tooth, choose small portions of sugar-free or low-sugar alternatives occasionally.

High-Sodium Foods: Reduce your intake of high-sodium foods such as processed meats, canned soups, salty snacks, and fast food, as they can increase blood pressure and the risk of heart disease. Choose fresh, whole foods and season meals with herbs and spices instead of salt.

Trans Fats: Avoid foods containing trans fats or hydrogenated oils, such as fried foods, commercial baked goods, and margarine. Trans fats can raise LDL cholesterol levels and increase the risk of heart disease, especially for individuals with diabetes.

White Bread and Refined Grains: Limit consumption of white bread, white rice, pasta, and other refined grains, as they are stripped of fiber and nutrients and can cause rapid spikes in blood sugar levels. Choose whole grains for better blood sugar control and sustained energy.

Full-Fat Dairy: While dairy products can be part of a healthy diabetes diet, opt for low-fat or non-fat options to reduce saturated fat intake and support heart health. Limit consumption of full-fat milk, cheese, and yogurt, which can contribute to elevated cholesterol levels.

Alcohol: Drink alcohol in moderation, if at all, as it can affect blood sugar levels and interfere with diabetes medication. Limit consumption to one drink per day for women and up to two drinks per day for men, and always consume alcohol with food to minimize its impact on blood sugar.

In conclusion, a balanced and nutritious diet plays a crucial role in managing diabetes and promoting optimum health for seniors over 50. By focusing on whole foods, lean proteins, healthy fats, and complex carbohydrates, while limiting processed foods, sugary treats, and unhealthy fats, individuals can effectively control blood sugar levels, prevent complications, and enjoy a vibrant and fulfilling life.

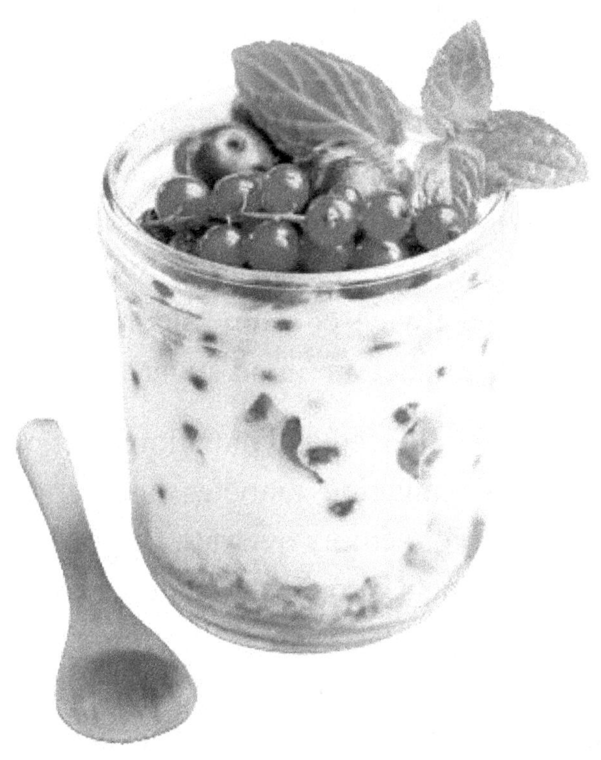

PART THREE:

Delicious diabetic breakfast recipes:

1. Veggie and Cheese Omelette

Ingredients:

- 2 eggs
- 1/4 cup diced bell peppers
- 1/4 cup diced tomatoes
- 1/4 cup diced onions
- 1/4 cup chopped spinach
- 1/4 cup shredded low-fat cheese
- Salt and pepper to taste
- 1 tsp olive oil

Instructions:

1. Heat olive oil in a non-stick skillet over medium heat.

2. In a bowl, beat eggs and season with salt and pepper.

3. Pour eggs into the skillet and let them cook for 1-2 minutes.

4. Sprinkle vegetables and cheese evenly over one half of the omelette.

5. Fold the other half of the omelette over the filling and cook for an additional 2-3 minutes, until the cheese is melted and the eggs are cooked through.

6. Serve hot with a side of whole grain toast or fresh fruit.

Servings: 1 Nutritional Value per serving:

- Calories: 250

- Protein: 20g

- Carbohydrates: 7g

- Fat: 15g

- Fiber: 2g

- Sodium: 300mg

Cooking Time: 10 minutes

2. Greek Yogurt Parfait

Ingredients:

- 1/2 cup plain Greek yogurt (low-fat or non-fat)
- 1/4 cup fresh berries (such as strawberries, blueberries, or raspberries)
- 1 tbsp chopped nuts (such as almonds or walnuts)
- 1 tbsp unsweetened coconut flakes
- 1 tsp honey or stevia (optional)

Instructions:

1. In a glass or bowl, layer Greek yogurt, fresh berries, chopped nuts, and coconut flakes.
2. Drizzle honey or sprinkle stevia over the top for sweetness, if desired.
3. Repeat layers if necessary.
4. Serve immediately or refrigerate for later.

Servings: 1 **Nutritional Value per serving:** Calories: 200, Protein: 18g, Carbohydrates: 15g, Fat: 8g, Fiber: 5g, Sodium: 50mg

Cooking Time: 5 minutes

3. Avocado Toast

Ingredients:

- 1 slice whole grain bread
- 1/2 ripe avocado, 1/2 tsp lemon juice
- Pinch of salt and pepper
- Optional toppings: sliced tomatoes, sprouts, boiled egg slices, or smoked salmon

Instructions:

1. Toast the whole grain bread until golden brown.
2. In a small bowl, mash the avocado with lemon juice, salt, and pepper.
3. Spread the mashed avocado evenly over the toast.
4. Top with desired toppings such as sliced tomatoes, sprouts, boiled egg slices, or smoked salmon.
5. Serve immediately.

Servings: 1 **Nutritional Value per serving:** Calories: 250, Protein: 7g, Carbohydrates: 20g, Fat: 15g, Fiber: 7g, Sodium: 150mg

Cooking Time: 5 minutes

Ingredients:

- 4 eggs

- 1/4 cup diced mushrooms

- 1/4 cup chopped spinach

- 1/4 cup diced onions

- 1/4 cup diced bell peppers

- Pinch of Salt and pepper to taste

- Cooking spray

Instructions:

1. Preheat the oven to 350°F (175°C). Grease a muffin tin with cooking spray.

2. In a bowl, beat eggs and season with salt and pepper.

3. Stir in diced mushrooms, chopped spinach, onions, and bell peppers.

4. Pour the egg mixture evenly into the muffin tin, filling each cup about three-quarters full.

5. Bake for 20-25 minutes, or until the egg muffins are set and lightly golden.

6. Allow the muffins to cool slightly before removing them from the tin.

7. Serve warm or store in an airtight container in the refrigerator for up to 3 days.

Servings: 2 (2 egg muffins per serving) **Nutritional Value per serving:**

- Calories: 150

- Protein: 12g

- Carbohydrates: 5g

- Fat: 9g

- Fiber: 2g

- Sodium: 200mg

Cooking Time: 25 minutes

5. Berry Protein Smoothie

Ingredients:

- 1/2 cup unsweetened almond milk
- 1/2 cup plain Greek yogurt (low-fat or non-fat)
- 1/2 cup mixed berries (such as strawberries, blueberries, and raspberries)
- 1 scoop vanilla protein powder (unsweetened)
- 1 tbsp chia seeds
- Ice cubes (optional)

Instructions:

1. In a blender, combine almond milk, Greek yogurt, mixed berries, protein powder, and chia seeds.

2. Blend until smooth and creamy, adding ice cubes if desired for a thicker consistency.

3. Pour into a glass and serve immediately.

Servings: 1 **Nutritional Value per serving:** Calories: 250, Protein: 25g, Carbohydrates: 20g, Fat: 8g, Fiber: 8g, Sodium: 150mg

Cooking Time: 5 minutes

Ingredients:

- 1/2 cup cooked quinoa
- 1/4 cup sliced almonds
- 1/4 cup diced apples
- 1/4 cup dried cranberries (unsweetened)
- 1/4 tsp cinnamon
- 1/4 cup unsweetened almond milk

Instructions:

1. In a bowl, combine cooked quinoa, sliced almonds, diced apples, dried cranberries, and cinnamon.

2. Pour unsweetened almond milk over the top and stir to combine.

3. Microwave the quinoa mixture for 1-2 minutes, or until heated through.

4. Serve hot and enjoy.

Servings: 1 **Nutritional Value per serving:** Calories: 300, Protein: 8g, Carbohydrates: 40g, Fat: 12g, Fiber: 6g, Sodium: 50mg

Cooking Time: 5 minutes

7. Chia Seed Pudding

Ingredients:

- 2 tbsp chia seeds

- 1/2 cup unsweetened almond milk

- 1/2 tsp vanilla extract

- 1 tsp honey or stevia (optional)

- Fresh fruit for topping (such as berries or sliced bananas)

- Nuts or seeds for topping (such as almonds or pumpkin seeds)

Instructions:

1. In a jar or bowl, combine chia seeds, almond milk, vanilla extract, and honey or stevia, if using.

2. Stir well to combine and ensure that the chia seeds are evenly distributed.

3. Refrigerate the mixture for at least 2 hours or overnight, stirring occasionally to prevent clumping.

4. Once the chia seeds have absorbed the liquid and formed a pudding-like consistency, remove from the refrigerator.

5. Serve topped with fresh fruit, nuts, or seeds for added flavor and texture.

Servings: 1 **Nutritional Value per serving:** Calories: 200, Protein: 6g, Carbohydrates: 20g, Fat: 10g, Fiber: 10g, Sodium: 50mg

Cooking Time: 5 minutes (plus chilling time)

8. Vegetable Breakfast Burrito

Ingredients:

- 1 whole grain tortilla
- 2 eggs, scrambled
- 1/4 cup diced bell peppers
- 1/4 cup diced onions
- 1/4 cup diced tomatoes
- 1/4 cup chopped spinach
- 1/4 cup shredded low-fat cheese
- Salsa or hot sauce for serving (optional)

Instructions:

1. Heat a non-stick skillet over medium heat.

2. Place the whole grain tortilla in the skillet and warm it for 1-2 minutes on each side.

3. In a separate pan, scramble the eggs until cooked through.

4. Fill the tortilla with scrambled eggs, diced bell peppers, onions, tomatoes, chopped spinach, and shredded cheese.

5. Roll up the tortilla to form a burrito.

6. Serve with salsa or hot sauce on the side, if desired.

Servings: 1 Nutritional Value per serving:

- Calories: 300

- Protein: 20g

- Carbohydrates: 25g

- Fat: 12g

- Fiber: 5g

- Sodium: 250mg

Cooking Time: 10 minutes

9. Banana Almond Butter Toast

Ingredients:

- 1 slice whole grain bread, toasted
- 1 tbsp almond butter (unsweetened)
- 1/2 banana, sliced
- 1 tsp honey or stevia (optional)

Instructions:

1. Spread almond butter evenly over the toasted whole grain bread.

2. Arrange sliced bananas on top of the almond butter.

3. Drizzle honey or sprinkle stevia over the bananas for sweetness, if desired.

4. Serve immediately.

Servings: 1 **Nutritional Value per serving:** Calories: 250, Protein: 7g, Carbohydrates: 30g, Fat: 12g, Fiber: 6g, Sodium: 150mg

Cooking Time: 5 minutes

Ingredients:

- 1 whole grain tortilla
- 2 eggs, scrambled
- 1/4 cup diced bell peppers
- 1/4 cup diced onions
- 1/4 cup diced tomatoes
- 1/4 cup chopped spinach
- Salt and pepper to taste
- Cooking spray

Instructions:

1. Heat a non-stick skillet over medium heat and coat with cooking spray.

2. Add diced bell peppers and onions to the skillet and sauté until softened.

3. Add diced tomatoes and chopped spinach to the skillet and cook until wilted.

4. Season with salt and pepper to taste.

5. In a separate pan, scramble the eggs until cooked through.

6. Warm the whole grain tortilla in the skillet for 1-2 minutes on each side.

7. Fill the tortilla with scrambled eggs and cooked vegetables.

8. Roll up the tortilla to form a wrap.

9. Serve immediately.

Servings: 1 Nutritional Value per serving:

- Calories: 300

- Protein: 20g

- Carbohydrates: 25g

- Fat: 12g

- Fiber: 5g

- Sodium: 250mg

Cooking Time: 15 minutes

Delicious diabetic salad recipes:

1. Mixed Green Salad with Grilled Chicken

Ingredients:

- 2 cups mixed greens (such as spinach, arugula, and romaine)

- 4 oz grilled chicken breast, sliced

- 1/4 cup cherry tomatoes, halved

- 1/4 cup cucumber, sliced

- 1/4 cup bell peppers, diced

- 1/4 cup shredded carrots

- 1 tbsp balsamic vinaigrette dressing (low-sodium)

Instructions:

1. In a large bowl, combine mixed greens, grilled chicken breast, cherry tomatoes, cucumber, bell peppers, and shredded carrots.

2. Drizzle balsamic vinaigrette dressing over the salad and toss to coat evenly.

3. Serve immediately.

Servings: 1 **Nutritional Value per serving:** Calories: 250, Protein: 30g, Carbohydrates: 10g, Fat: 10g, Fiber: 4g, Sodium: 200mg

Preparation Time: 15 minutes

2. Quinoa and Black Bean Salad

Ingredients:

- 1/2 cup cooked quinoa

- 1/4 cup black beans, drained and rinsed

- 1/4 cup corn kernels (fresh or frozen, thawed)

- 1/4 cup diced tomatoes

- 1/4 cup diced red onions

- 1/4 cup chopped cilantro

- Juice of 1 lime

- Salt and pepper to taste

Instructions:

1. In a large bowl, combine cooked quinoa, black beans, corn kernels, diced tomatoes, diced red onions, and chopped cilantro.

2. Squeeze fresh lime juice over the salad and season with salt and pepper to taste.

3. Toss to combine all ingredients evenly.

4. Serve chilled or at room temperature.

Servings: 1 **Nutritional Value per serving:** Calories: 300, Protein: 10g, Carbohydrates: 45g, Fat: 5g, Fiber: 8g, Sodium: 150mg

Preparation Time: 20 minutes

3. Mediterranean Chickpea Salad

Ingredients:

- 1/2 cup canned chickpeas, drained and rinsed

- 1/4 cup cucumber, diced

- 1/4 cup cherry tomatoes, halved

- 1/4 cup Kalamata olives, pitted and halved

- 1/4 cup red onion, thinly sliced

- 2 tbsp crumbled feta cheese (low-fat)

- 1 tbsp extra virgin olive oil

- 1 tbsp lemon juice

- 1 tsp dried oregano

- Pinch of Salt and pepper to taste

Instructions:

1. In a large bowl, combine chickpeas, cucumber, cherry tomatoes, Kalamata olives, red onion, and crumbled feta cheese.

2. Drizzle extra virgin olive oil and lemon juice over the salad.

3. Sprinkle dried oregano, salt, and pepper over the salad and toss gently to combine.

4. Serve immediately or refrigerate for later.

Servings: 1 Nutritional Value per serving:

- Calories: 300

- Protein: 10g

- Carbohydrates: 25g

- Fat: 15g

- Fiber: 8g

- Sodium: 300mg

Preparation Time: 15 minutes

Ingredients:

- 1/2 cup canned white beans, drained and rinsed
- 2 oz canned tuna in water, drained
- 1/4 cup cherry tomatoes, halved
- 1/4 cup cucumber, diced
- 1/4 cup red bell peppers, diced
- 1 tbsp red onion, finely chopped
- 1 tbsp fresh parsley, chopped
- 1 tbsp lemon juice
- 1 tsp Dijon mustard
- Pinch of Salt and pepper to taste

Instructions:

1. In a large bowl, combine white beans, canned tuna, cherry tomatoes, cucumber, red bell peppers, red onion, and fresh parsley.

2. In a small bowl, whisk together lemon juice, Dijon mustard, salt, and pepper to make the dressing.

3. Pour the dressing over the salad and toss gently to combine.

4. Serve chilled or at room temperature.

Servings: 1 Nutritional Value per serving:

- Calories: 250

- Protein: 25g

- Carbohydrates: 20g

- Fat: 8g

- Fiber: 6g

- Sodium: 300mg

Preparation Time: 15 minutes

5. Spinach and Strawberry Salad

Ingredients:

- 2 cups baby spinach leaves
- 1/2 cup sliced strawberries
- 1/4 cup sliced almonds
- 1/4 cup crumbled feta cheese (low-fat)
- 1 tbsp balsamic vinegar
- 1 tbsp extra virgin olive oil
- 1 tsp honey or stevia (optional)

Instructions:

1. In a large bowl, combine baby spinach leaves, sliced strawberries, sliced almonds, and crumbled feta cheese.

2. In a small bowl, whisk together balsamic vinegar, extra virgin olive oil, and honey or stevia, if using, to make the dressing.

3. Drizzle the dressing over the salad and toss gently to coat.

4. Serve immediately.

Servings: 1 **Nutritional Value per serving:**
Calories: 200, Protein: 8g, Carbohydrates: 15g, Fat:
12g, Fiber: 6g, Sodium: 200mg

Preparation Time: 10 minutes

6. Asian Edamame Salad

Ingredients:

- 1 cup shelled edamame, cooked

- 1/2 cup shredded cabbage

- 1/4 cup shredded carrots

- 1/4 cup diced red bell peppers

- 2 tbsp sliced green onions

- 1 tbsp sesame seeds

- 1 tbsp low-sodium soy sauce

- 1 tbsp rice vinegar

- 1 tsp sesame oil

- 1/2 tsp grated ginger

- 1/2 tsp honey or stevia (optional)

Instructions:

1. In a large bowl, combine shelled edamame, shredded cabbage, shredded carrots, diced red bell peppers, sliced green onions, and sesame seeds.

2. In a small bowl, whisk together low-sodium soy sauce, rice vinegar, sesame oil, grated ginger, and honey or stevia, if using, to make the dressing.

3. Pour the dressing over the salad and toss gently to coat.

4. Serve chilled or at room temperature.

Servings: 1 Nutritional Value per serving:

- Calories: 250

- Protein: 15g

- Carbohydrates: 20g

- Fat: 10g

- Fiber: 8g

- Sodium: 300mg

Preparation Time: 15 minutes

7. Caprese Salad

Ingredients:

- 1 cup cherry tomatoes, halved
- 1/2 cup fresh mozzarella balls
- 1/4 cup fresh basil leaves
- 1 tbsp extra virgin olive oil
- 1 tbsp balsamic glaze
- Pinch of Salt and pepper to taste

Instructions:

1. In a large bowl, combine cherry tomatoes, fresh mozzarella balls, and fresh basil leaves.
2. Drizzle extra virgin olive oil and balsamic glaze over the salad.
3. Season with salt and pepper to taste.
4. Toss gently to combine.
5. Serve immediately.

Servings: 1 **Nutritional Value per serving:** Calories: 300, Protein: 15g, Carbohydrates: 10g, Fat: 20g, Fiber: 2g, Sodium: 300mg

Preparation Time: 10 minutes

8. Kale and Quinoa Salad

Ingredients:

- 2 cups chopped kale leaves
- 1/2 cup cooked quinoa
- 1/4 cup diced cucumber
- 1/4 cup diced red bell peppers
- 1/4 cup diced carrots
- 2 tbsp sliced almonds
- 1 tbsp lemon juice
- 1 tbsp extra virgin olive oil
- Pinch of Salt and pepper to taste

Instructions:

1. In a large bowl, massage chopped kale leaves with lemon juice and extra virgin olive oil for a few minutes to soften.

2. Add cooked quinoa, diced cucumber, diced red bell peppers, diced carrots, and sliced almonds to the bowl.

3. Season with salt and pepper to taste.

4. Toss gently to combine.

5. Serve chilled or at room temperature.

Servings: 1 **Nutritional Value per serving:** Calories: 250, Protein: 10g, Carbohydrates: 30g, Fat: 10g, Fiber: 8g, Sodium: 200mg

Preparation Time: 15 minutes

9. Beet and Goat Cheese Salad

Ingredients:

- 1 cup cooked and diced beets

- 2 cups mixed greens (such as arugula and spinach)

- 1/4 cup crumbled goat cheese

- 2 tbsp chopped walnuts

- 1 tbsp balsamic vinegar

- 1 tbsp extra virgin olive oil

- Pinch of Salt and pepper to taste

Instructions:

1. In a large bowl, combine cooked and diced beets, mixed greens, crumbled goat cheese, and chopped walnuts.

2. Drizzle balsamic vinegar and extra virgin olive oil over the salad.

3. Season with salt and pepper to taste.

4. Toss gently to combine.

5. Serve immediately.

Servings: 1 Nutritional Value per serving:

- Calories: 300

- Protein: 10g

- Carbohydrates: 20g

- Fat: 20g

- Fiber: 5g

- Sodium: 300mg

Preparation Time: 15 minutes

10. Cucumber and Avocado Salad

Ingredients:

- 1 large cucumber, sliced
- 1/2 avocado, diced
- 1/4 cup diced red onion
- 1/4 cup cherry tomatoes, halved
- 2 tbsp chopped cilantro
- Juice of 1 lime
- 1 tbsp extra virgin olive oil
- Pinch of Salt and pepper to taste

Instructions:

1. In a large bowl, combine sliced cucumber, diced avocado, diced red onion, cherry tomatoes, and chopped cilantro.
2. Squeeze fresh lime juice over the salad and drizzle with extra virgin olive oil.
3. Season with salt and pepper to taste.
4. Toss gently to combine.

5. Serve chilled or at room temperature.

Servings: 1 Nutritional Value per serving:

- Calories: 250

- Protein: 5g

- Carbohydrates: 20g

- Fat: 15g

- Fiber: 8g

- Sodium: 200mg

Preparation Time: 10 minutes

These 10 delicious diabetic salad recipes offer a variety of flavors, textures, and nutritional benefits to enjoy while managing diabetes and promoting overall health. Each recipe is carefully crafted to be low in sugar, low in carbs, low in sodium, and low in fat, making them suitable for individuals with diabetes, heart disease, and kidney concerns. Incorporate these salads into your meal plan for a satisfying and nutritious dining experience.

Delicious diabetic main dish recipes:

1. Grilled Salmon with Asparagus

Ingredients:

- 2 salmon fillets (6 oz each)
- 1 bunch asparagus, trimmed
- 2 tbsp olive oil
- 1 lemon, sliced
- Pinch of Salt and pepper to taste

Instructions:

1. Preheat grill to medium-high heat.

2. Brush salmon fillets and asparagus with olive oil and season with salt and pepper.

3. Place salmon fillets and lemon slices on the grill and cook for 4-5 minutes per side, or until fish is cooked through and flakes easily with a fork.

4. Grill asparagus for 3-4 minutes, or until tender-crisp.

5. Serve grilled salmon and asparagus with lemon slices on the side.

Servings: 2 **Nutritional Value per serving:** Calories: 350, Protein: 30g, Carbohydrates: 10g, Fat: 20g, Fiber: 4g, Sodium: 100mg

Cooking Time: 15 minutes

2. Turkey and Vegetable Stir-Fry

Ingredients:

- 8 oz lean ground turkey
- 2 cups mixed vegetables (such as bell peppers, broccoli, carrots, and snap peas)
- 2 cloves garlic, minced
- 2 tbsp low-sodium soy sauce
- 1 tbsp sesame oil
- 1 tsp ginger, grated
- 2 green onions, sliced
- Cooked brown rice or quinoa for serving

Instructions:

1. Heat sesame oil in a large skillet over medium heat.

2. Add ground turkey and cook until browned, breaking it apart with a spoon.

3. Add mixed vegetables, garlic, ginger, and soy sauce to the skillet.

4. Stir-fry for 5-6 minutes, or until vegetables are tender.

5. Serve turkey and vegetable stir-fry over cooked brown rice or quinoa.

6. Garnish with sliced green onions before serving.

Servings: 2 Nutritional Value per serving:

- Calories: 300

- Protein: 25g

- Carbohydrates: 20g

- Fat: 12g

- Fiber: 6g

- Sodium: 300mg

Cooking Time: 20 minutes

3. Baked Chicken with Roasted Vegetables

Ingredients:

- 2 boneless, skinless chicken breasts

- 2 cups mixed vegetables (such as carrots, potatoes, and Brussels sprouts)

- 2 tbsp olive oil

- 2 cloves garlic, minced

- 1 tsp dried herbs (such as thyme or rosemary)

- Pinch of Salt and pepper to taste

Instructions:

1. Preheat oven to 400°F (200°C).

2. Place chicken breasts on a baking sheet lined with parchment paper.

3. In a bowl, toss mixed vegetables with olive oil, minced garlic, dried herbs, salt, and pepper.

4. Arrange vegetables around the chicken on the baking sheet.

5. Bake for 25-30 minutes, or until chicken is cooked through and vegetables are tender.

6. Serve baked chicken with roasted vegetables hot from the oven.

Servings: 2 Nutritional Value per serving:

- Calories: 300

- Protein: 30g

- Carbohydrates: 15g

- Fat: 12g

- Fiber: 5g

- Sodium: 150mg

Cooking Time: 30 minutes

4. Shrimp and Vegetable Stir-Fry

Ingredients:

- 8 oz shrimp, peeled and deveined
- 2 cups mixed vegetables (such as bell peppers, snap peas, and mushrooms)
- 2 cloves garlic, minced
- 2 tbsp low-sodium soy sauce
- 1 tbsp olive oil
- 1 tsp sesame seeds
- Cooked brown rice or quinoa for serving

Instructions:

1. Heat olive oil in a large skillet over medium heat.
2. Add shrimp and cook for 2-3 minutes per side, or until pink and opaque.
3. Remove shrimp from the skillet and set aside.
4. In the same skillet, add mixed vegetables and minced garlic.

5. Stir-fry for 4-5 minutes, or until vegetables are tender-crisp.

6. Return shrimp to the skillet and add low-sodium soy sauce.

7. Cook for an additional 1-2 minutes, stirring to coat everything evenly.

8. Serve shrimp and vegetable stir-fry over cooked brown rice or quinoa.

9. Garnish with sesame seeds before serving.

Servings: 2 Nutritional Value per serving:

- Calories: 250

- Protein: 20g

- Carbohydrates: 15g

- Fat: 10g

- Fiber: 4g

- Sodium: 200mg

Cooking Time: 20 minutes

5. Baked Cod with Lemon and Herbs

Ingredients:

- 2 cod fillets (6 oz each)

- 1 lemon, sliced

- 2 tbsp fresh parsley, chopped

- 1 tbsp olive oil

- 2 cloves garlic, minced

- Pinch of Salt and pepper to taste

Instructions:

1. Preheat oven to 400°F (200°C).

2. Place cod fillets on a baking sheet lined with parchment paper.

3. Drizzle olive oil over the cod fillets and sprinkle minced garlic, chopped parsley, salt, and pepper on top.

4. Place lemon slices on top of the cod fillets.

5. Bake for 15-20 minutes, or until fish is cooked through and flakes easily with a fork.

6. Serve baked cod with lemon and herbs hot from the oven.

Servings: 2 **Nutritional Value per serving:** Calories: 200, Protein: 25g, Carbohydrates: 5g, Fat: 8g, Fiber: 2g, Sodium: 100mg

Cooking Time: 20 minutes

6. Vegetable and Tofu Stir-Fry

Ingredients:

- 1 block firm tofu, pressed and cubed
- 2 cups mixed vegetables (such as broccoli, bell peppers, and snow peas)
- 2 cloves garlic, minced
- 2 tbsp low-sodium soy sauce
- 1 tbsp sesame oil
- 1 tsp cornstarch mixed with 2 tbsp water
- Cooked brown rice or quinoa for serving

Instructions:

1. Heat sesame oil in a large skillet over medium heat.

2. Add cubed tofu to the skillet and cook until golden brown on all sides.

3. Remove tofu from the skillet and set aside.

4. In the same skillet, add mixed vegetables and minced garlic.

5. Stir-fry for 4-5 minutes, or until vegetables are tender-crisp.

6. Return tofu to the skillet and add low-sodium soy sauce.

7. Stir in cornstarch mixture and cook for an additional 1-2 minutes, until the sauce has thickened.

8. Serve vegetable and tofu stir-fry over cooked brown rice or quinoa.

Servings: 2 **Nutritional Value per serving:** Calories: 250, Protein: 15g, Carbohydrates: 20g, Fat: 10g, Fiber: 6g, Sodium: 300mg

Cooking Time: 25 minutes

Ingredients:

- 8 oz lean ground turkey

- 1 bell pepper, cut into chunks

- 1 zucchini, sliced

- 1 onion, cut into chunks

- 1/4 cup low-sodium teriyaki sauce

- Wooden skewers, soaked in water

Instructions:

1. Preheat grill to medium-high heat.

2. Divide ground turkey into equal portions and shape each portion onto wooden skewers.

3. Thread bell pepper chunks, zucchini slices, and onion chunks onto separate skewers.

4. Grill turkey and vegetable skewers for 8-10 minutes, turning occasionally, or until turkey is cooked through and vegetables are tender.

5. Brush skewers with low-sodium teriyaki sauce during the last few minutes of cooking.

6. Serve turkey and vegetable skewers hot from the grill.

Servings: 2 **Nutritional Value per serving:** Calories: 300, Protein: 25g, Carbohydrates: 15g, Fat: 12g, Fiber: 5g, Sodium: 200mg

Cooking Time: 15 minutes

8. Lentil and Vegetable Soup

Ingredients:

- 1 cup dry green lentils

- 4 cups low-sodium vegetable broth

- 2 cups mixed vegetables (such as carrots, celery, and tomatoes)

- 1 onion, diced

- 2 cloves garlic, minced

- 1 tsp dried thyme

- Pinch of Salt and pepper to taste

Instructions:

1. In a large pot, combine dry green lentils, low-sodium vegetable broth, mixed vegetables, diced onion, minced garlic, and dried thyme.

2. Bring the soup to a boil over medium-high heat.

3. Reduce heat to low, cover, and simmer for 25-30 minutes, or until lentils and vegetables are tender.

4. Season with salt and pepper to taste.

5. Serve lentil and vegetable soup hot, garnished with fresh herbs if desired.

Servings: 4 Nutritional Value per serving:

- Calories: 250

- Protein: 15g

- Carbohydrates: 40g

- Fat: 5g

- Fiber: 12g

- Sodium: 200mg

Cooking Time: 35 minutes

9. Chicken and Vegetable Skillet

Ingredients:

- 2 boneless, skinless chicken breasts

- 2 cups mixed vegetables (such as bell peppers, broccoli, and carrots)

- 2 cloves garlic, minced

- 2 tbsp olive oil

- 1/4 cup low-sodium chicken broth

- 1 tbsp lemon juice

- Pinch of Salt and pepper to taste

Instructions:

1. Season chicken breasts with salt and pepper on both sides.

2. Heat olive oil in a large skillet over medium-high heat.

3. Add chicken breasts to the skillet and cook for 5-6 minutes per side, or until golden brown and cooked through.

4. Remove chicken from the skillet and set aside.

5. In the same skillet, add mixed vegetables and minced garlic.

6. Stir-fry for 4-5 minutes, or until vegetables are tender-crisp.

7. Return chicken to the skillet and add low-sodium chicken broth and lemon juice.

8. Cook for an additional 2-3 minutes, or until heated through.

9. Serve chicken and vegetable skillet hot from the skillet.

Servings: 2 Nutritional Value per serving:

- Calories: 300

- Protein: 30g

- Carbohydrates: 15g

- Fat: 12g

- Fiber: 5g

- Sodium: 200mg

Cooking Time: 20 minutes

Ingredients:

- 1 eggplant, diced

- 1 can chickpeas, drained and rinsed

- 1 onion, diced

- 2 cloves garlic, minced

- 1 tbsp curry powder

- 1 cup low-sodium vegetable broth

- 1/2 cup canned coconut milk (unsweetened)

- 2 tbsp olive oil

- Fresh cilantro for garnish

- Cooked brown rice for serving

Instructions:

1. Heat olive oil in a large pot over medium heat.

2. Add diced eggplant, diced onion, and minced garlic to the pot.

3. Cook for 5-6 minutes, or until vegetables are softened.

4. Stir in curry powder and cook for an additional 1-2 minutes.

5. Add drained chickpeas, low-sodium vegetable broth, and canned coconut milk to the pot.

6. Bring the mixture to a simmer and cook for 15-20 minutes, or until eggplant is tender and curry has thickened.

7. Season with salt and pepper to taste.

8. Serve eggplant and chickpea curry hot, garnished with fresh cilantro and served over cooked brown rice.

Servings: 4 Nutritional Value per serving:

- Calories: 300
- Protein: 10g
- Carbohydrates: 30g
- Fat: 15g
- Fiber: 8g
- Sodium: 150mg

Cooking Time: 30 minutes

Delicious diabetic seafood recipes:

1. Grilled Lemon Garlic Shrimp

Ingredients:

- 1 lb large shrimp, peeled and deveined
- 2 cloves garlic, minced
- 2 tbsp olive oil
- 1 lemon, juiced and zested
- Salt and pepper to taste
- Skewers (if using wooden, soak in water for 30 minutes)

Instructions:

1. Preheat grill to medium-high heat.
2. In a bowl, combine minced garlic, olive oil, lemon juice, lemon zest, salt, and pepper.
3. Add shrimp to the bowl and toss to coat evenly.
4. Thread shrimp onto skewers if using.
5. Grill shrimp for 2-3 minutes per side, or until pink and cooked through.
6. Serve hot with a squeeze of lemon juice.

Servings: 4 **Nutritional Value per serving:** Calories: 150, Protein: 20g, Carbohydrates: 2g, Fat: 7g, Fiber: 0g, Sodium: 150mg

Cooking Time: 10 minutes

2. Baked Salmon with Dill Sauce

Ingredients:

- 4 salmon fillets (6 oz each)
- 2 tbsp chopped fresh dill
- 2 cloves garlic, minced
- 2 tbsp Greek yogurt (low-fat)
- 1 lemon, juiced
- Pinch of Salt and pepper to taste

Instructions:

1. Preheat oven to 375°F (190°C).

2. In a small bowl, mix together chopped dill, minced garlic, Greek yogurt, lemon juice, salt, and pepper.

3. Place salmon fillets on a baking sheet lined with parchment paper.

4. Spread the dill sauce over the salmon fillets.

5. Bake for 12-15 minutes, or until salmon is cooked through and flakes easily with a fork.

6. Serve hot with additional lemon wedges if desired.

Servings: 4 Nutritional Value per serving:

- Calories: 250

- Protein: 30g

- Carbohydrates: 2g

- Fat: 12g

- Fiber: 0g

- Sodium: 100mg

Cooking Time: 15 minutes

3. Garlic Herb Grilled Swordfish

Ingredients:

- 4 swordfish steaks (6 oz each)
- 2 cloves garlic, minced
- 2 tbsp chopped fresh parsley
- 2 tbsp olive oil
- 1 lemon, juiced
- Pinch of Salt and pepper to taste

Instructions:

1. Preheat grill to medium-high heat.
2. In a small bowl, mix together minced garlic, chopped parsley, olive oil, lemon juice, salt, and pepper.
3. Brush both sides of the swordfish steaks with the garlic herb mixture.
4. Grill swordfish steaks for 4-5 minutes per side, or until fish is cooked through and opaque.
5. Serve hot with additional lemon wedges if desired.

Servings: 4 **Nutritional Value per serving:** Calories: 300, Protein: 25g, Carbohydrates: 1g, Fat: 15g, Fiber: 0g, Sodium: 100mg

Cooking Time: 10 minutes

4. Lemon Herb Baked Cod

Ingredients:

- 4 cod fillets (6 oz each)
- 2 tbsp chopped fresh parsley
- 2 tbsp chopped fresh dill
- 2 cloves garlic, minced
- 2 tbsp olive oil
- 1 lemon, juiced and zested

Instructions:

1. Preheat oven to 375°F (190°C).

2. In a small bowl, mix together chopped parsley, chopped dill, minced garlic, olive oil, lemon juice, lemon zest, salt, and pepper.

3. Place cod fillets on a baking sheet lined with parchment paper.

4. Spread the lemon herb mixture over the cod fillets.

5. Bake for 12-15 minutes, or until cod is cooked through and flakes easily with a fork.

6. Serve hot with additional lemon wedges if desired.

Servings: 4 Nutritional Value per serving:

- Calories: 200

- Protein: 25g

- Carbohydrates: 1g

- Fat: 10g

- Fiber: 0g

- Sodium: 100mg

Cooking Time: 15 minutes

5. Spicy Grilled Shrimp Skewers

Ingredients:

- 1 lb large shrimp, peeled and deveined
- 2 cloves garlic, minced
- 2 tbsp olive oil
- 1 tbsp paprika
- 1 tsp cayenne pepper
- 1 tsp dried oregano
- Salt and pepper to taste
- Skewers (if using wooden, soak in water for 30 minutes)

Instructions:

1. Preheat grill to medium-high heat.
2. In a bowl, combine minced garlic, olive oil, paprika, cayenne pepper, dried oregano, salt, and pepper.
3. Add shrimp to the bowl and toss to coat evenly.
4. Thread shrimp onto skewers if using.
5. Grill shrimp for 2-3 minutes per side, or until pink and cooked through.

6. Serve hot with a squeeze of lemon juice.

Servings: 4 **Nutritional Value per serving:** Calories: 150, Protein: 20g, Carbohydrates: 2g, Fat: 7g, Fiber: 0g, Sodium: 150mg

Cooking Time: 10 minutes

6. Herb Crusted Baked Tilapia

Ingredients:

- 4 tilapia fillets (6 oz each)

- 1/4 cup almond meal

- 2 tbsp chopped fresh parsley

- 2 tbsp grated Parmesan cheese

- 2 cloves garlic, minced

- 2 tbsp olive oil

Instructions:

1. Preheat oven to 400°F (200°C).

2. In a small bowl, mix together almond meal, chopped parsley, grated Parmesan cheese, minced garlic, olive oil, salt, and pepper.

3. Place tilapia fillets on a baking sheet lined with parchment paper.

4. Press the herb mixture onto the top of each tilapia fillet.

5. Bake for 12-15 minutes, or until tilapia is cooked through and flakes easily with a fork.

6. Serve hot with a wedge of lemon if desired.

Servings: 4 Nutritional Value per serving:

- Calories: 200

- Protein: 25g

- Carbohydrates: 3g

- Fat: 9g

- Fiber: 1g

- Sodium: 150mg

Cooking Time: 15 minutes

7. Garlic Butter Lemon Scallops

Ingredients:

- 1 lb sea scallops
- 2 cloves garlic, minced
- 2 tbsp unsalted butter
- 1 lemon, juiced and zested
- 2 tbsp chopped fresh parsley

Instructions:

1. Pat dry the sea scallops with paper towels and season with salt and pepper.

2. Heat butter in a large skillet over medium-high heat.

3. Add minced garlic to the skillet and cook until fragrant.

4. Add sea scallops to the skillet and cook for 2-3 minutes per side, or until golden brown and cooked through.

5. Drizzle lemon juice over the scallops and sprinkle with lemon zest and chopped parsley.

6. Serve hot with additional lemon wedges if desired.

Servings: 4 Nutritional Value per serving:

- Calories: 150

- Protein: 20g

- Carbohydrates: 2g

- Fat: 7g

- Fiber: 0g

- Sodium: 200mg

Cooking Time: 10 minutes

8. Cajun Grilled Catfish

Ingredients:

- 4 catfish fillets (6 oz each)
- 2 tbsp Cajun seasoning
- 2 tbsp olive oil
- 1 lemon, juiced
- Pinch of Salt to taste

Instructions:

1. Preheat grill to medium-high heat.
2. Rub Cajun seasoning and olive oil over both sides of the catfish fillets.
3. Season with salt to taste.
4. Grill catfish fillets for 4-5 minutes per side, or until fish is cooked through and flakes easily with a fork.
5. Drizzle lemon juice over the grilled catfish before serving.

Servings: 4 **Nutritional Value per serving:** Calories: 250, Protein: 30g, Carbohydrates: 2g, Fat: 12g, Fiber: 0g, Sodium: 200mg

Cooking Time: 10 minutes

9. Mediterranean Baked Halibut

Ingredients:

- 4 halibut fillets (6 oz each)
- 2 tbsp olive oil
- 2 cloves garlic, minced
- 1 tsp dried oregano
- 1/2 tsp dried thyme
- 1/2 tsp dried basil
- 1/2 cup cherry tomatoes, halved
- 1/4 cup Kalamata olives, pitted and sliced
- Pinch of Salt and pepper to taste

Instructions:

1. Preheat oven to 375°F (190°C).

2. In a small bowl, mix together olive oil, minced garlic, dried oregano, dried thyme, dried basil, salt, and pepper.

3. Place halibut fillets on a baking sheet lined with parchment paper.

4. Brush the olive oil mixture over the halibut fillets.

5. Scatter cherry tomatoes and Kalamata olives around the halibut fillets.

6. Bake for 12-15 minutes, or until halibut is cooked through and flakes easily with a fork.

7. Serve hot with a side of steamed vegetables.

Servings: 4 Nutritional Value per serving:

- Calories: 250

- Protein: 30g

- Carbohydrates: 4g

- Fat: 12g

- Fiber: 1g

- Sodium: 200mg

Cooking Time: 15 minutes

10. Coconut Lime Shrimp Curry

Ingredients:

- 1 lb large shrimp, peeled and deveined
- 1 can coconut milk (unsweetened)
- 2 cloves garlic, minced
- 1 onion, diced
- 1 red bell pepper, sliced
- 1 tbsp curry powder
- 1 lime, juiced and zested
- 2 tbsp chopped fresh cilantro
- Pinch of Salt and pepper to taste

Instructions:

1. In a large skillet, heat coconut milk over medium heat.
2. Add minced garlic, diced onion, and sliced red bell pepper to the skillet.
3. Cook until vegetables are softened.
4. Stir in curry powder, lime juice, and lime zest.

5. Add shrimp to the skillet and cook for 3-4 minutes, or until shrimp is pink and cooked through.

6. Season with salt and pepper to taste.

7. Serve hot, garnished with chopped fresh cilantro.

Servings: 4 **Nutritional Value per serving:** Calories: 200 , Protein: 20g, Carbohydrates: 5g, Fat: 10g, Fiber: 2g, Sodium: 150mg

Cooking Time: 20 minutes

These delicious diabetic recipes offer a variety of flavors, textures, and nutritional benefits to enjoy while managing diabetes and promoting overall health. Each recipe is carefully crafted to be low in sugar, low in carbs, low in sodium, and low in fat, making them suitable for individuals with diabetes, heart disease, and kidney concerns. Incorporate these Anti-inflammatory food dishes into your meal plan for a satisfying and nutritious dining experience.

CONCLUSION

The "Diabetes Diet Cookbook for Seniors Over 50" offers a comprehensive array of delicious, nutritious, and diabetes-friendly recipes tailored specifically for the unique dietary needs of older adults. Through careful selection of natural, low-sugar, low-carb, low-sodium, and low-fat ingredients, these recipes not only aim to manage diabetes but also promote overall health and well-being. From hearty main dishes to refreshing salads and delectable seafood options, each recipe is crafted with meticulous attention to flavor, texture, and nutritional balance.

By embracing the recipes in this cookbook, seniors over 50 can take proactive steps towards managing their diabetes naturally while enhancing their overall health. With an abundance of anti-inflammatory ingredients and scientifically proven recipes, this cookbook serves as a valuable tool for individuals seeking to improve their quality of life through mindful eating habits.

Remember, managing diabetes is not just about restricting certain foods but rather about making informed choices and enjoying a varied and flavorful diet. By incorporating the recipes from this cookbook into your daily routine, you are not only nourishing your body but also nourishing your soul. Embrace the journey towards better health with each delicious bite, knowing that every meal brings you one step closer to a happier, healthier, and more vibrant life. Take charge of your health today and savor the joys of good food and good health for years to come.

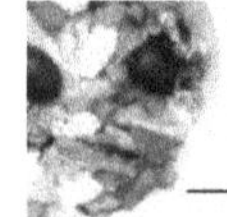

MEAL PLANNER

DATE:

	BREAKFAST	LUNCH	DINNER	SHOPPING LIST
MON				
TUES				
WED				
THURS				
FRI				
SAT				
SUN				

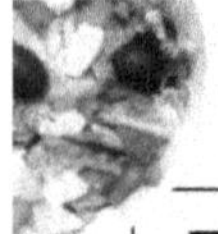 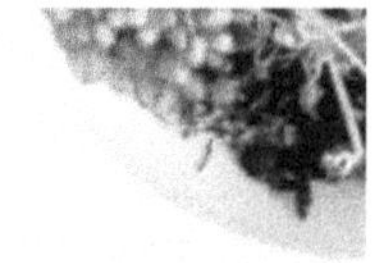

MEAL PLANNER

DATE:

	BREAKFAST	LUNCH	DINNER	SHOPPING LIST
MON				
TUES				
WED				
THURS				
FRI				
SAT				
SUN				

MEAL PLANNER

DATE:

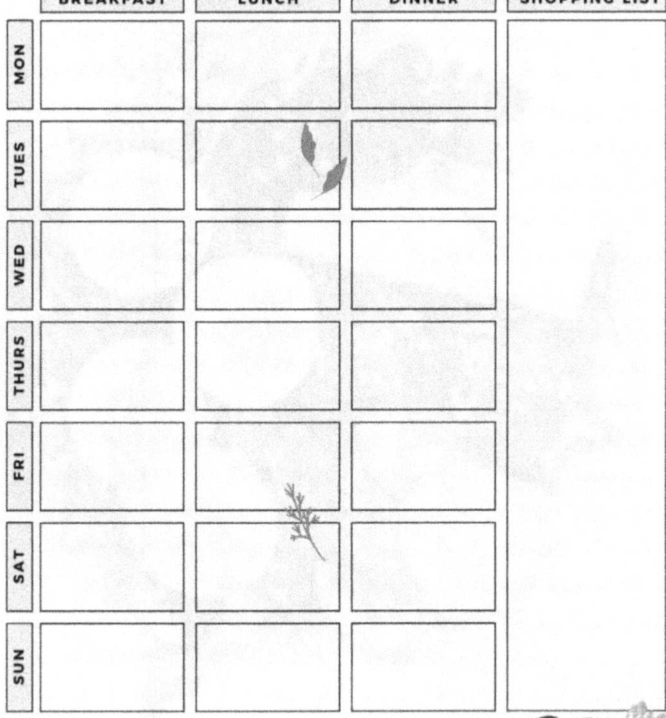

	BREAKFAST	LUNCH	DINNER	SHOPPING LIST
MON				
TUES				
WED				
THURS				
FRI				
SAT				
SUN				

MEAL PLANNER

DATE:

	BREAKFAST	LUNCH	DINNER	SHOPPING LIST
MON				
TUES				
WED				
THURS				
FRI				
SAT				
SUN				

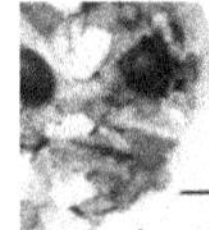

MEAL PLANNER

DATE:

	BREAKFAST	LUNCH	DINNER	SHOPPING LIST
MON				
TUES				
WED				
THURS				
FRI				
SAT				
SUN				

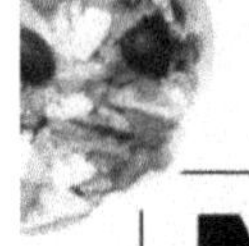

MEAL PLANNER

DATE: ___________

	BREAKFAST	LUNCH	DINNER	SHOPPING LIST
MON				
TUES				
WED				
THURS				
FRI				
SAT				
SUN				

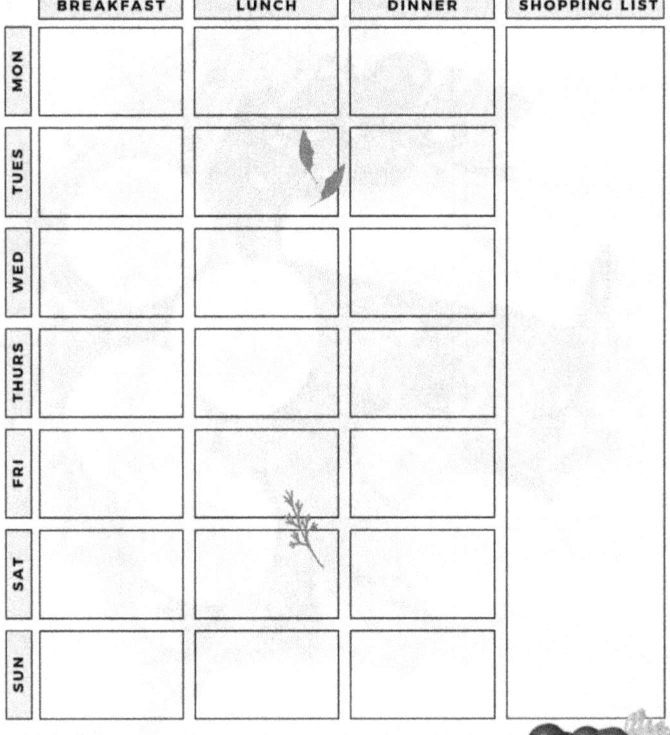

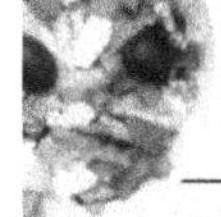

MEAL PLANNER

DATE: _______________

	BREAKFAST	LUNCH	DINNER	SHOPPING LIST
MON				
TUES				
WED				
THURS				
FRI				
SAT				
SUN				

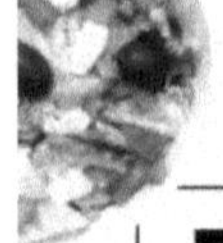

MEAL PLANNER

DATE:

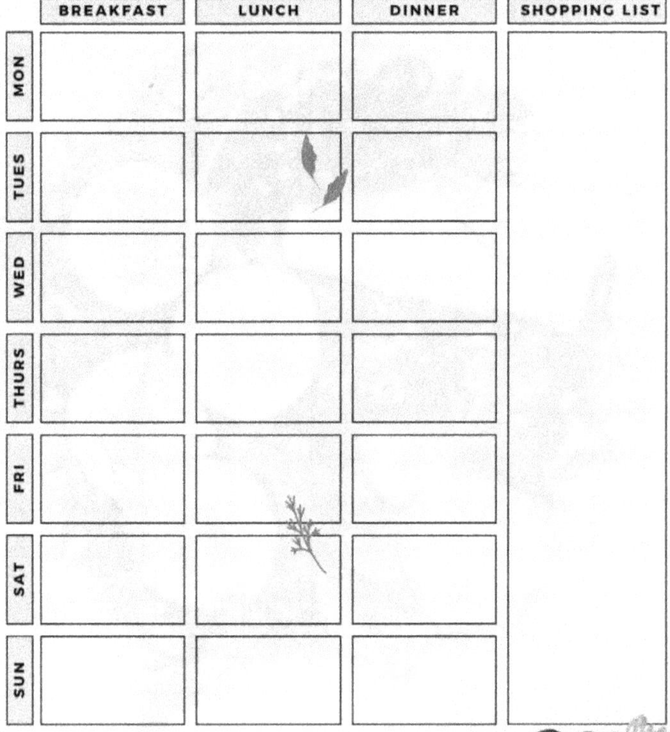

	BREAKFAST	LUNCH	DINNER	SHOPPING LIST
MON				
TUES				
WED				
THURS				
FRI				
SAT				
SUN				

MEAL PLANNER

DATE:

	BREAKFAST	LUNCH	DINNER	SHOPPING LIST
MON				
TUES				
WED				
THURS				
FRI				
SAT				
SUN				

MEAL PLANNER

DATE:

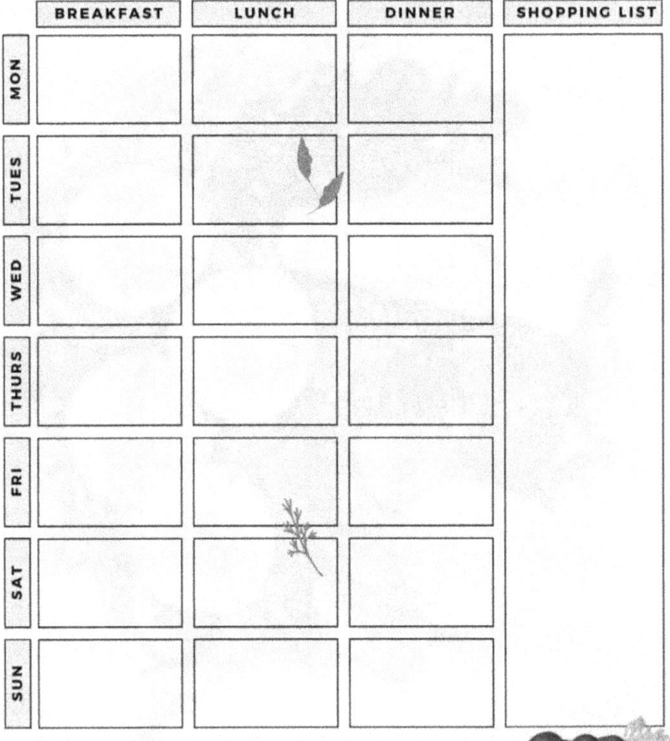

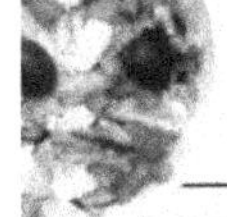

MEAL PLANNER

DATE:

	BREAKFAST	LUNCH	DINNER	SHOPPING LIST
MON				
TUES				
WED				
THURS				
FRI				
SAT				
SUN				

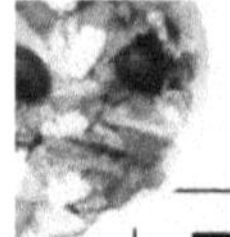

MEAL PLANNER

DATE:

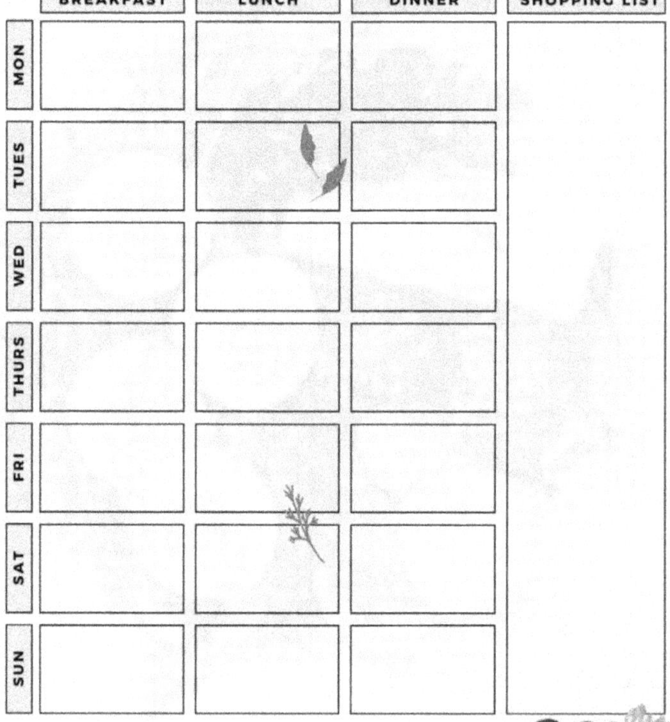

	BREAKFAST	LUNCH	DINNER	SHOPPING LIST
MON				
TUES				
WED				
THURS				
FRI				
SAT				
SUN				

www.ingramcontent.com/pod-product-compliance
Lightning Source LLC
Chambersburg PA
CBHW070818280726
48660CB00016B/2058